THE SUPERCHARGED METABOLIC CONFUSION DIET FOR ENDOMORPHS

Lose weight effortlessly with tasty recipes, a list of healthy foods, a cookbook, and a 30-day meal plan. This guide will empower you to outsmart your body and achieve a healthier weight.

Vincent John Walker

Disclaimer

This publication is designed to provide competent and reliable information regarding the subject covered. However, the views expressed in this publication are those of the author alone, and should not be taken as expert instruction or professional advice. The reader is responsible for his or her actions. The author hereby disclaims any responsibility or liability whatsoever that is incurred from the use or application of the contents of this publication by the purchaser of the reader. The purchaser or reader is hereby responsible for his or her actions.

Copyright © 2024

Table of Contents

Introduction

Step into "The Supercharged Metabolic Confusion Diet for Endomorphs," a unique and personalized path to achieving better health and fitness designed especially for those with an endomorphic body type. This comprehensive diet plan is carefully crafted to tap into the concept of metabolic confusion, offering a practical and flexible framework to support endomorphs as they embark on their transformative journey to a healthier lifestyle.

Endomorphs, who typically have a propensity to store excess body fat and a curvier physique, encounter distinct challenges in weight management and fitness achievement. The Supercharged Metabolic Confusion Diet recognizes and addresses these challenges, providing an individualized roadmap to boost metabolism, elevate energy levels, and facilitate sustainable weight loss.

This program isn't a one-size-fits-all remedy. Instead, it embraces the uniqueness of endomorphs, understanding that what works for one body type may not be equally effective for another. By incorporating the principles of metabolic confusion, the diet introduces deliberate variations in calorie intake, macronutrient distribution, and meal timing. This intentional diversity prevents the body from getting accustomed to a fixed routine, ensuring a stimulated metabolism and promoting efficient calorie burning.

On this journey, you'll explore a variety of nutrient-rich foods, delightful recipes, and practical meal plans tailored to meet the specific needs of endomorphs. From protein-rich meals to wise carbohydrate choices and healthy fats, each aspect of this diet is crafted to support your metabolic well-being, manage cravings, and encourage a sustainable and enjoyable approach to nutrition.

Beyond dietary advice, "The Supercharged Metabolic Confusion Diet for Endomorphs" integrates valuable insights into lifestyle considerations, exercise routines, and mindset strategies that complement the dietary plan. This holistic approach aims to equip individuals with the knowledge and tools needed to make enduring changes, fostering a positive relationship with food and promoting overall well-being.

Embark on this transformative journey with confidence, recognizing that this diet plan is more than just about shedding pounds – it's about embracing a lifestyle that aligns with your distinctive body type and personal goals. Welcome to an innovative approach to nutrition that acknowledges and celebrates the diversity of bodies – welcome to "The Supercharged Metabolic Confusion Diet for Endomorphs." Your journey toward a healthier, more energized you start right here.

Understanding Your Endomorph Body Type

For decades, the concept of body types has enthralled academics, fitness enthusiasts, and those seeking change. Endomorphs, who are known for their inclination to store body fat fast, have a hereditary tendency that may make weight management difficult. This chapter delves into the complexity of the endomorph body type, looking at the genetic and physiological factors that contribute to their unique metabolic response.

The Role of Metabolism in Weight Management

Metabolism is the engine that powers our bodies' complex biochemical processes. Understanding how metabolism influences weight management is critical to understanding this material. We examine the physics behind basal metabolic rate (BMR), thermogenesis, and the factors that may aid or hinder an endomorph's calorie-burning processes. Understanding the connection between metabolism and weight gives a solid foundation for the transformational path ahead.

What is the Metabolic Confusion Diet?

The Metabolic Confusion Diet is more than just a fad diet. It is a scientifically backed and intentional strategy for feeding that takes into account endomorph variations. By using the power of metabolic confusion, this diet claims to fire up your metabolism, reduce plateaus, and support long-term weight loss. This chapter explains the principles of the diet, showing how cyclical macronutrient change and feeding timing may increase fat loss and energy levels.

As you begin your investigation of the Metabolic Confusion Diet for Endomorphs, keep in mind that each person's journey is as unique as their genetic makeup. This book will be your companion while you work toward your health and fitness objectives, giving guidance, instruction, and support. Remember that transformation is about accepting the process, learning about your body, and developing a positive relationship with food, exercise, and yourself.

Endomorph Metabolism: The Science Behind It

Genetics and Body Composition

The complicated link between inheritance and body composition is a hot issue in biology, medicine, and fitness. Our genetic make-up has a significant impact on aspects of our physical appearance, metabolism, and inclination to gain or lose weight. Understanding the complex relationship between genetics and body composition is crucial for understanding why individuals have diverse body types, responses to diet and exercise, and susceptibility to certain health issues.

Genetic Influence on Body Composition:

Genetics substantially influences body composition, which refers to the distribution of fat, muscle, bone, and other tissues in the body. Variables such as basal metabolic rate (BMR), fat storage, muscle growth, and hunger control are all regulated by different genes. These genetic factors may determine whether a person is an endomorph, ectomorph, or mesomorph—three common body types characterized based on how they gain or lose weight and their general form.

Fat Storage and Genetics:

Genetic variations may influence how our bodies store and transport fat. Some individuals, according to their genetic makeup, may naturally retain excess fat in certain areas, such as the hips, thighs, or belly. This inclination to retain fat may have an impact on body shape and the weight-control challenges that various body types face.

Muscle Growth and Genetics:

Genetics also have a role in an individual's capacity to build muscle and strength. Specific genes regulate muscle fiber composition, muscle responsiveness to exercise, and muscle protein synthesis efficiency. This explains why some individuals seem to grow muscle faster than others, and why some types of physical activity may be more effective for certain people.

Appetite Regulation and Genetic Variability:

Appetite and hunger are complex processes regulated by several hormones and neurotransmitters. Genetic variations may influence how our bodies react to these signals, impacting hunger, fullness, and food choices. Individuals with certain genetic profiles may have a higher or reduced propensity to feel full after meals, influencing their eating patterns and, as a consequence, their body composition.

Adapting to Genetic Predispositions:

It is important to understand that although genetics provide the foundation, they do not determine your destiny. Genetic predispositions may impact body composition, but lifestyle factors such as diet, exercise, sleep, stress management, and environmental influences all play a role. A well-planned diet and exercise routine may help individuals work with their genetic tendencies to achieve their desired body composition goals.

Factors Influencing Hormones and Metabolism

Metabolism is the sum of all biochemical operations that occur inside the body to maintain life. It entails the transformation of food into energy, the development and repair of tissues, and the control of several physiological functions. Hormones, being powerful messengers, play a critical role in metabolic control. Knowledge of how our bodies regulate energy, weight, and overall health requires an understanding of the relationship between metabolism and hormonal factors.

Hormones' Role in Metabolism:

Hormones are chemical messengers produced by the many glands of the endocrine system. These molecules circulate in the bloodstream, where they bind to specific receptors on target cells, causing specific responses. Hormones affect metabolism by controlling how the body consumes and stores energy, how it reacts to stress, and how it regulates food and wants.

The Basal Metabolic Rate and Thyroid Hormones:

Thyroid hormones, which are produced by the thyroid gland, are crucial in metabolic control. The thyroid hormones thyroxine (T4) and triiodothyronine (T3) influence the basal metabolic rate (BMR), which is the amount of energy consumed by the body at rest to support fundamental functions. Thyroid hormone abnormalities may induce changes in BMR, altering the body's ability to burn calories.

Controlling Blood Sugar Using Insulin:

Insulin, which is produced by the pancreas, is necessary for blood sugar regulation. Carbohydrates are broken down into glucose, which enters the bloodstream after consumption. Insulin promotes glucose transport into cells for utilization as energy or storage. Insulin sensitivity or resistance may cause high blood sugar levels and weight gain, especially around the belly.

Appetite Control using Leptin and Ghrelin:

Leptin and ghrelin are hunger and satiety hormones, respectively. Leptin, which is produced by fat cells, tells the brain that the body has enough stored energy, influencing feelings of fullness. Ghrelin, which is produced in the stomach, stimulates appetite. The imbalance of these hormones may affect the body's ability to sense hunger and fullness, perhaps leading to overeating or undereating.

Cortisol and Stress Response:

Cortisol, sometimes known as "stress hormone," is a hormone produced by the adrenal glands in response to stress. While stress is important for survival, chronic stress may result in elevated cortisol levels, which can impair metabolism. Cortisol levels that are higher than usual have been related to an increase in belly fat storage, as well as changes in appetite and nutritional choices.

Sex Hormones and Metabolism:

Men's and women's metabolisms are affected differently by sex hormones such as estrogen and testosterone. Estrogen is linked to fat storage and distribution, while testosterone is linked to muscle development and energy expenditure. Hormonal changes at different stages of life, such as puberty, pregnancy, and menopause, may have an impact on metabolism and body composition.

Balanced Hormones for Optimal Metabolism:

A healthy metabolism is reliant on hormonal balance. Lifestyle factors such as eating, exercise, sleep, and stress management may all have an impact on hormone levels. A nutrient-dense diet encourages hormone production and regulation. Regular physical exercise may improve insulin sensitivity and support healthy hormonal responses. Prioritizing sleep and managing stress might help to avoid hormonal imbalances that can hinder metabolism and weight management.

Endomorph Weight Gain and Loss Influencing Factors

Endomorphs have a natural tendency to store body fat more readily than other body types. This proclivity may make weight management more challenging, but understanding the variables that drive weight gain and loss in endomorphs may empower people to make informed choices and successfully adopt weight-management techniques.

Genetic Disease Predisposition:

An individual's body type, metabolism, and how their body reacts to varied foods and activities are all influenced by genetics. Endomorphs are predisposed genetically to have higher body fat and a slower metabolism. While genetics have a part, they do not decide your destiny; your lifestyle choices may have a significant impact.

Endomorphs usually have a lower basal metabolic rate (BMR), which is the amount of energy expended by the body while it is at rest. This may be attributed to genetics, hormone influences, and body composition. Endomorphs with slower metabolisms may burn fewer calories at rest, making weight gain easier if their calorie intake is not well managed.

Fat Storage Patterns:

Endomorphs tend to gain fat faster, especially in certain areas such as the hips, thighs, and abdomen. This may make it tough to lose body fat in certain locations. Understanding these patterns may help in the formulation of exercise and diet strategies to reduce fat in these areas.

Elements of Hormones:

Hormones such as cortisol and insulin may impact endomorph weight gain and loss. Higher cortisol levels, which are commonly associated with stress, may lead to the buildup of belly fat. Insulin sensitivity, or how well the body reacts to insulin, may affect how well endomorphs consume carbohydrates and keep blood sugar levels stable.

Dietary Alternatives:

Endomorphs may be more prone to storing additional calories as fat. This means that their dietary choices are crucial for weight control. They need a diet that is balanced in macronutrients and provides the necessary number of calories to sustain their activity level. Avoiding processed carbohydrates and sweets may help reduce blood sugar spikes and crashes.

Physical Activity:

While endomorphs may struggle with weight control due to their genetics, regular physical activity is still a vital part of achieving and maintaining a healthy weight. Exercise raises energy expenditure, enhances metabolic rate, and promotes muscle growth, all of which may increase calorie burning even when you're not doing anything.

Individual Variation:

It's important to remember that everyone is different, and even within the same body type, there may be significant disparities.

Some endomorphs may have faster metabolisms and unique fat distribution patterns than others. The difficult equation of weight regulation includes age, gender, lifestyle choices, and overall health.

Metabolic Confusion Diet Principles

Cycling Macronutrients for the Best Results

Cycling macronutrients is a diet that includes varying carbohydrate, protein, and fat intake on different days or at different times. This technique is often used to optimize nutrient consumption, promote different objectives (such as fat loss or muscle growth), and prevent the body from reacting to a consistent intake. Endomorphs who struggle with weight management may benefit from cycling macronutrients.

- **Cycling macronutrients** may assist in preventing metabolic adaptation, a phenomenon in which the body becomes used to a given calorie intake and slows its metabolism. By adjusting your macronutrient ratios regularly, you can keep your metabolism active and more sensitive to changes in food consumption.

- **Managing Insulin Levels:** Endomorphs may be more prone to insulin resistance, which may lead to blood sugar increases and fat gain. Macronutrient cycling, especially carbohydrate cycling, may help manage insulin levels and enhance sensitivity, which are both beneficial for weight reduction.

- **Increasing Fat Loss:** Cycling carbohydrates, specifically reducing carbohydrate intake on certain days, may increase fat loss by encouraging the body to rely more on stored fat for energy. This may lead to a calorie deficit while preserving muscle mass.

- **Support for muscle growth:** Protein intake is necessary for muscle mending and development. Cycling protein intake may boost muscle protein synthesis and offer the amino acids needed for repair and development on days when you concentrate on resistance exercise.

- **Plateaus:** Changing your macronutrient intake regularly helps your body from plateauing, which is a common occurrence in which weight loss or muscle building stops due to adaptation. Macronutrient cycling keeps your body guessing and prevents complacency.

- **Adapting to Lifestyle Changes:** Macronutrient cycling enables you to customize your diet to your amount of activity, objectives, and lifestyle changes. This adaptability may make the method more sustainable in the long term.

- **Cycling macronutrients** may help balance hormones such as insulin and leptin, which control appetite, fat storage, and metabolism. This may result in improved appetite control and fat loss.

Techniques for Cycling Macronutrients

There are many techniques for macronutrient cycling, and each may be adapted to individual tastes and objectives. The following are some of the most common approaches:

- Carb cycling is the practice of alternating days of higher carbohydrate consumption with days of lower carbohydrate consumption. This is extremely beneficial for fat loss.
- Calorie cycling is the practice of varying total calorie intake on different days while keeping relatively identical macronutrient ratios. This approach may help to avoid metabolic adaptation.
- Protein cycling refers to varying protein intake based on activity level and objectives. Protein intake on training days is increased to support muscle building and recovery.
- Refeed Days: Include higher carbohydrate days strategically to replenish glycogen stores and avoid metabolic slowdown.
- Intermittent fasting is characterized by a period of fasting followed by a period of normal or increased calorie and macronutrient intake.

Meal Frequency and Timing Are Important

Meal frequency and timing are crucial in optimizing metabolism, energy levels, and overall health. Endomorphs, who may struggle with weight control, may benefit from sensible meal timing and frequency in achieving their health and fitness goals.

- Blood Sugar Levels: Eating at regular intervals helps to manage blood sugar levels by reducing spikes and crashes, which may lead to cravings and overeating. Endomorphs need stable blood sugar levels to regulate their insulin response and prevent excessive fat storage.

- Eating at regular intervals helps to avoid extreme hunger, which may lead to overeating or poor food choices. Endomorphs, who tend to overeat, may benefit from planned meals and snacks to help them regulate their appetite.

- Improving Nutrient Utilization: Timing meals strategically may increase the body's capacity to absorb and use nutrients. Protein and carbohydrates, for example, help in muscle repair and glycogen replenishment before and after exercise.

- Increasing Metabolism: Eating frequent, well-balanced meals signals to the body that it is obtaining a steady supply of energy. This may assist in keeping the body from entering "starvation mode," which causes metabolism to slow down to save energy.

- Avoiding Overeating: Eating short meals throughout the day might keep the digestive system from being overwhelmed by big meals. This may assist those who digest slowly to prevent discomfort and bloating.

- Eating at regular intervals provides a continuous flow of energy, preventing energy dumps and helping you maintain focus and productivity throughout the day.

- Weight Control: Eating at regular intervals may help regulate calorie intake and prevent excessive fat storage in endomorphs, who have a propensity to store fat more rapidly.

- Muscle Mass Maintenance: A high protein intake increases muscle protein synthesis, which contributes to the preservation and development of lean muscle mass. This is especially important for endomorphs who want to reduce weight since muscle burns more calories at rest than fat.

Strategies for Meal Timing and Frequency

Here are some suggestions for meal planning and frequency:

- *Meals:* Aim for three main meals and two to three snacks each day. This reduces the amount of time between meals, which may lead to overeating.

- *Breakfast with Protein:* Start your day with a protein-rich breakfast. This may help with desire control and provide long-lasting energy.

- *Pre- and post-workout nutrition:* Before working out, fuel your body with a combination of carbohydrates and protein. After exercise, consume protein and carbohydrates to assist recovery and replenish glycogen levels.

- *Carbohydrate Distribution:* Spread out your carbohydrate consumption evenly throughout the day. Large carbohydrate-heavy meals, particularly in the evening, should be avoided.

- *Mindful Eating:* Pay attention to your body's hunger and fullness cues. Do not push yourself to eat if you are not hungry, but do not wait till you are.

- *Hydration:* Drink lots of water throughout the day to stay hydrated, which may also help you regulate your appetite.

- *Individualized Approach:* Remember that everyone's requirements and preferences differ. Experiment with different meal times and frequency patterns to see which works best for your body and lifestyle.

Personalization of Endomorph Diet

Endomorph diet customization comprises tailoring nutritional solutions to their unique genetic propensity and weight management difficulties. Endomorphs may eat in a way that supports their goals while also promoting long-term health and wellbeing by understanding their metabolism, body composition, and any hormonal imbalances.

- Endomorphs may be more sensitive to carbohydrates, especially refined sugars, and meals with a high glycemic index, may cause blood sugar spikes. Consume complex carbohydrates, such as whole grains, vegetables, and legumes, in moderation. Carbohydrates may be strategically arranged around exercises to aid with energy and recovery.

- Protein is required for the maintenance of lean muscle mass, metabolic support, and satiety. Include lean protein sources including poultry, fish, lean meats, eggs, dairy, and plant-based proteins in your meals and snacks. Protein intake is especially important before and after exercise.

- Avocados, almonds, seeds, olive oil, and fatty seafood are all good sources of healthful fats. Fats bring satisfaction while also aiding hormone production and general health. Because fats are abundant in calories, keep your portion sizes in check.

- Meal Timing: Spread out your meals and snacks throughout the day to prevent excessive hunger and overeating. Include protein and complex carbohydrates in each meal to help manage blood sugar levels and boost energy levels.

- Eat less processed and highly refined meals, which may contribute to weight gain and insulin resistance. Choose whole, nutrient-dense meals strong in vitamins and minerals.

- Drink enough water throughout the day to aid digestion, metabolism, and overall health. Staying hydrated might also help you regulate your hunger.

- Meal Control: Keep an eye on your meal proportions to avoid ingesting too many calories. Use visual cues such as your palm or a smaller dish to determine appropriate portions.

- While calorie counting isn't always necessary, understanding your anticipated calorie needs might help you avoid overeating. Aim for a little calorie deficit to lose weight.

- Strength Training: Strength training should be done regularly to grow and maintain lean muscle mass. Muscle burns more calories while it is at rest, which may help with weight loss.

- Regular cardiovascular exercise should be included in your daily routine to enhance your overall health and energy expenditure. To make exercising more fun, choose activities that you like.

- Mindful Eating: Be mindful of symptoms of hunger and fullness. Mindful eating allows you to savor your meals, avoid emotional eating, and make sensible food choices.

- Stress Management: Long-term stress may cause weight gain and hormonal imbalances. Stress-reduction techniques such as meditation, yoga, deep breathing, and enjoyable hobbies should be incorporated.

- Seek Professional Assistance: Speak with a qualified dietitian or nutritionist who specializes in weight management and endomorph nutrition. They may provide specialized guidance and assistance based on your needs and goals.

How to Begin the Metabolic Confusion Diet

Setting Specific Goals and Expectations

Setting clear objectives and expectations is critical for endomorph success on the Metabolic Confusion Diet. Setting well-defined aims and appropriate expectations will help you remain motivated, analyze your progress, and make educated choices. Here's a checklist to help you outline the objectives and expectations of your change.

- ***Determine Your Goals:*** Begin by identifying your objectives. Do you want to reduce weight, gain muscle, have more energy, or improve your overall health? Having specific objectives provides your efforts with emphasis and direction.

- ***Be specific:*** Make your objectives tangible and specific. Instead of stating, "I want to lose weight," define how much and when you want to lose it.

- ***Set Realistic Expectations:*** While huge dreams are great, make sure your objectives are feasible. Unrealistic expectations may lead to disappointment and discontent.

- ***Break Down Your Goals:*** Break down your larger goal into smaller, more doable steps. If you want to lose 20 pounds in six months, set monthly goals and develop a plan for each month.

- ***Focus on Non-Scale Gains:*** While weight reduction is the primary goal, consider non-scale gains such as more energy, better sleep, enhanced fitness levels, and increased happiness. These victories provide a thorough picture of your progress.

- ***Create a timetable:*** Establish a timetable for achieving your objectives. A timeline adds urgency and helps you remain on track.

- ***Be adaptable:*** Life is unpredictable, and progress may not always be linear. Be open to changing your objectives and tactics as required without getting discouraged.

- ***Document Your Success:*** You may track your progress using measurements, photographs, fitness tests, and writing. Tracking your development holds you responsible and provides you with a visual representation of your progress.

- ***Celebrate Milestones:*** Whether modest or significant, acknowledge your achievements along the way. Recognizing achievements boosts motivation and confirms your commitment.

- ***Visualize Success:*** Visualize yourself achieving your goals. Visualizing success may help you establish a positive mindset and increase your confidence in your ability to succeed.

- ***Be patient:*** It takes time for change to take place. Avoid comparing your achievement to others', and remember that consistency is key.

- ***Monitor potential stumbling blocks:*** Anticipate potential stumbling blocks and obstacles. Create strategies for dealing with them and keeping on track.

- ***Maintain a Positive Attitude:*** Practice positive thinking and self-talk. Be kind to yourself, particularly when you are facing setbacks or plateaus.

- ***Seek Assistance:*** Discuss your goals with a friend, family member, or accountability partner who can encourage and inspire you.

- ***Review frequently:*** Evaluate your objectives and progress regularly. Are you on the correct path? Do your goals need to be revised? Regular assessments keep you on pace to meet your objectives.

Examining Your Current Diet and Lifestyle

Before making any dietary or lifestyle changes, you should assess your current habits and activities. This evaluation provides critical information about where you are and helps you to make informed choices about how to tailor the Metabolic Confusion Diet for Endomorphs to your needs. Here's a step-by-step guide to assessing your current diet and lifestyle:

- ***Keep a Food Journal:*** Over a few days, keep note of everything you eat and drink, including portion sizes and meal times. This gives you a better understanding of your eating patterns and helps you to find areas for improvement.

- ***Examine Your Food Record:*** Examine your food record to determine the macronutrient balance (carbohydrates, proteins, and fats) in your diet. Do you get a variety of nutrients from different sources?

- ***Keep Snacking Behaviors Tracked:*** Keep track of your snacking habits. Do you munch haphazardly, out of boredom, or in response to emotions? Identifying triggers may help you make better judgments.

- ***Monitor your hydration:*** How much water do you drink each day? Hydration is essential for overall health and may influence energy levels and metabolism.

- ***Examine Meal Proportions:*** Match portion sizes to your hunger and satiety cues. Do you eat till you're full, or do you overeat?

- ***Consider Food Options:*** Consider the kind of meals you often consume. Are you consuming largely whole, nutrient-dense meals, or mostly processed, high-calorie foods?

- ***Consider Meal Timing:*** Consider when you eat your meals and snacks. Do you eat at regular intervals or do you go long periods between meals?

- ***Monitor Physical Activity:*** Think about your current exercise routine. How often do you exercise, and what kind of exercises do you prefer?

- ***Examine Your Stress Levels:*** Examine your stress levels and how you handle stress. Chronic stress may have an impact on eating habits and weight management.

- ***Examine Sleep Patterns:*** Think about your sleeping habits. Do you get enough rejuvenating sleep? Sleep deprivation has been shown to affect metabolism and hunger regulation.

- ***Recognize Emotional Eating:*** Do you eat in response to negative emotions such as stress, boredom, or sadness? Recognizing emotional eating tendencies may aid in the development of good coping techniques.

- ***Monitor Your Energy Levels:*** Throughout the day, keep track of your energy levels. Do you experience regular energy slumps or fatigue?

- ***Examine Supplements:*** If you utilize supplements, assess their efficacy and need. Consult with a healthcare professional to verify that your supplement regimen is following your goals.

- ***Seek Professional Help:*** Visit a trained dietitian or nutritionist for a thorough examination of your diet and lifestyle. They may give tailored suggestions based on your individual needs and goals.

- ***Set Priorities:*** Based on your evaluation, determine which areas of change you want to concentrate on. Prioritize these features as you begin to create the Metabolic Confusion Diet for endomorphs.

Creating a Pleasant Environment

For the Metabolic Confusion Diet for Endomorphs to be successful, a supportive environment is required. Surrounding yourself with positive influences and establishing a successful atmosphere may have a significant effect on your ability to maintain healthy habits and accomplish your goals. Here's how to create a happy atmosphere:

- ***Determine Your Intentions:*** Determine your goals and motives for beginning the Metabolic Confusion Diet. A clear sense of purpose can help you stay motivated and focused.

- ***Educate Your Inner Circle:*** Talk about your goals with close friends, family members, or a supportive spouse. Inform them of your dietary choices so they may provide support and assist you in avoiding unintentional temptations.

- ***Meal Preparation and Planning:*** Make time for meal planning and preparation. When you have healthful meals and snacks on hand, you are less likely to make bad eating choices when you are hungry.

- ***Keep Nutrient-Dense Meals on Hand:*** Keep nutrient-dense foods on hand that are compatible with the Metabolic

Confusion Diet. This makes it simple to make healthy choices while cooking or snacking.

- *Limit Trigger Foods:* Keep trigger foods to a minimum in your household (things that are difficult to resist). If you have them, keep them concealed or in hard-to-reach places.

- *Create a Workout Space:* Create a workout space at home, even if it's only a little place for bodyweight exercises. A designated location encourages regular physical activity.

- *Schedule Regular Workouts:* Make time in your schedule for exercise as if it were an essential appointment. Consistency is important, and having a pattern in place makes it easier to stick to it.

- *Select a Workout Buddy:* If possible, choose a workout companion who shares your fitness goals. Working out with a partner enhances accountability and may make exercise more enjoyable.

- *Unplug from Negative Influences:* Limit your exposure to messages in the media or on social media regarding bad or unrealistic body image. Follow accounts that promote body positivity, health, and a balanced lifestyle.

- *Create Positive Visual Reminders:* Put motivational quotes, images, or your goals in visible places like your refrigerator, bathroom mirror, or computer screen.

- ***Mindful Eating Environment:*** Practice mindful eating by dining in a place free of distractions like screens or work. This may allow you to fully savor and appreciate your food.

- ***Stay Hydrated:*** Always have a water bottle nearby to promote ongoing hydration.

- ***Maintain a Journal to Document Your Thoughts, Feelings, and Development:*** Maintain a journal to document your thoughts, feelings, and progress. This may both inspire and help you spot patterns and challenges.

- ***Reward Yourself:*** Make a system of rewards for achieving objectives. Non-food rewards that relate to your interests and beliefs are an excellent way to reward yourself.

Metabolic Reset Phase 1

The duration and purpose of the Reset Phase

Endomorphs on the Metabolic Confusion Diet must complete the reset phase. It is the foundation of the eating strategy and aids your body in preparing for the subsequent stages. The length and purpose of the reset phase are important factors in its effectiveness.

Duration: Typically, the reset phase lasts one to two weeks. This initial session is designed to help your body adjust to changes in macronutrient intake, stabilize blood sugar levels, and reset your metabolism. The duration will be determined by your preferences, objectives, and the specific recommendations of your healthcare expert or nutritionist.

Purpose:

The following are the key aims of the reset phase:

- ***Metabolic Adaptation:*** The body adapts to consistent calorie and macronutrient ingestion. The reset phase diversifies your metabolism and prevents it from becoming extremely effective at using certain foods. This helps to prevent plateaus and promotes long-term fat loss.

- ***Blood Sugar Stabilization:*** If you've been consuming a lot of refined carbohydrates, the reset phase will assist you in re-establishing appropriate blood sugar levels. This may aid in the reduction of cravings, the enhancement of fullness, and the improvement of insulin sensitivity.

- ***While the body has inherent detoxifying skills,*** the reset phase may be considered as a way to reduce reliance on processed foods, sweets, and unhealthy fats. This might lead to better digestion and overall health.

- ***Reduced Inflammation:*** By temporarily reducing inflammatory foods, you may experience reduced bloating, improved skin health, and less water retention.

- ***Psychological transfer:*** The reset phase represents the transition from previous eating behaviors to the principles of the Metabolic Confusion Diet. It permits you to psychologically prepare for the more structured stages to come.

Approaching the Phase of Reset:

Throughout the reset phase, you'll focus on substantial, nutrient-dense meals, balanced macronutrient ratios, and portion control. Here's how you do it:

- Whole Foods: Include in your diet lean meats, vegetables, fruits, whole grains, nuts, seeds, and healthy fats.

- Meals that are well-balanced in terms of protein, carbohydrates, and fats are ideal. This helps to keep blood sugar levels stable and increases fullness.

- Reduce or eliminate your use of processed meals, sugary snacks, and high-calorie drinks.

- Stay hydrated by drinking lots of water throughout the day.

- Conscious Eating: Teach yourself to recognize hunger and fullness cues. Avoid distractions when eating.

- Meal Control: Keep track of your meal quantities and avoid overeating.

While you'll be making better choices during this phase, avoid harsh limitations or major calorie deficits.

Foods that Endomorphs should consume when following the Metabolic Confusion Diet

During the various stages of the Metabolic Confusion Diet for endomorphs, the following foods are examples of nutrient-dense selections that might help you achieve your goals:

Proteins:

- Lean meats (chicken, turkey, lean cuts of beef or pork)
- Fish (salmon, trout, tuna)
- Eggs
- Greek yogurt
- Cottage cheese
- Tofu
- Legumes (beans, lentils, chickpeas)

Carbohydrates:

- Whole grains (quinoa, brown rice, oats, whole wheat)
- Fruits (berries, apples, oranges, bananas)
- Vegetables (leafy greens, broccoli, cauliflower, peppers)
- Sweet potatoes
- Legumes (black beans, kidney beans)
- Lentils

Fats:

- Avocado
- Nuts (almonds, walnuts, pistachios)
- Seeds (chia seeds, flaxseeds, pumpkin seeds)
- Olive oil
- Fatty fish (salmon, mackerel, sardines)

Dairy and Alternatives:

- Greek yogurt (plain, unsweetened)
- Cottage cheese (low-fat)
- Unsweetened almond milk, coconut milk, or other plant-based milk

Snacks:

- Fresh fruit
- Raw vegetables with hummus
- Greek yogurt with berries

- Handful of nuts

- Rice cakes with almond butter

Beverages:

- Water

- Herbal teas

- Black coffee (in moderation)

- Unsweetened herbal-infused water

Foods to Avoid or Limit:

While certain items should be consumed in moderation or avoided entirely, keep in mind that balance and moderation are fundamental concepts of the Metabolic Confusion Diet. Avoid or limit:

- ***Processed foods*** often have extra sugars, harmful fats, and unnatural ingredients.

- ***Sugary Snacks:*** Sugary snacks such as candy, pastries, sugary cereals, and sweetened drinks may cause blood sugar increases and fat accumulation.

- ***Trans Fats:*** Trans fat-rich foods, such as fried and packaged snacks, are unhealthy.

- ***Highly Refined Carbohydrates:*** Avoid white bread, white rice, and sugary cereals.

- ***Sugary Beverages:*** Sodas, energy drinks, and sugary juices may all contribute to calorie overload.

- ***Excessive alcohol*** use should be avoided since it may interfere with weight reduction and metabolic health.
- ***Excessive Salty Foods:*** Excessive salt consumption may cause water retention and bloating.
  Unhealthy Fats: Limit your intake of deep-fried meals and saturated fat-rich foods.

30-Day Meal Plans

Day 1:

- **Breakfast:** Scrambled eggs with spinach and whole-grain toast
- **Lunch:** Grilled chicken salad with mixed greens and colorful vegetables
- **Dinner:** Baked salmon with quinoa and steamed broccoli
- **Snack:** Greek yogurt with berries

Day 2:

- **Breakfast:** Greek yogurt parfait with fresh fruit and chia seeds
- **Lunch:** Lentil soup with whole-grain crackers
- **Dinner:** Stir-fried tofu with mixed vegetables and brown rice
- **Snack:** Handful of almonds

Day 3:

- **Breakfast:** Omelette with tomatoes, peppers, and feta cheese
- **Lunch:** Turkey and avocado wrap with whole wheat tortilla
- **Dinner:** Grilled shrimp with sweet potato wedges and sautéed spinach
- **Snack:** Fresh apple slices with a tablespoon of almond butter

Day 4:

- **Breakfast:** Cottage cheese and pineapple smoothie
- **Lunch:** Quinoa salad with black beans, corn, and diced tomatoes
- **Dinner:** Baked chicken breast with roasted Brussels sprouts and quinoa
- **Snack:** Handful of walnuts

Day 5:

- **Breakfast:** Whole-grain oatmeal with sliced bananas and chia seeds
- **Lunch:** Chickpea and vegetable curry with brown rice
- **Dinner:** Grilled trout with lemon, steamed asparagus, and sweet potato mash
- **Snack:** Raw vegetables with hummus

Day 6:

- **Breakfast:** Smoothie with unsweetened almond milk, mixed berries, and protein powder
- **Lunch:** Egg salad lettuce wraps with cherry tomatoes
- **Dinner:** Lean beef stir-fry with broccoli and whole wheat noodles
- **Snack:** Cottage cheese with sliced peaches

Day 7:

- **Breakfast:** Avocado toast on whole-grain bread with poached eggs
- **Lunch:** Tuna salad with mixed greens, cucumbers, and whole-grain croutons
- **Dinner:** Baked cod with quinoa and roasted cauliflower
- **Snack:** Handful of pistachios

Day 8:

- **Breakfast:** Whole-grain waffles with fresh berries and Greek yogurt
- **Lunch:** Chicken and vegetable kebabs with whole-wheat couscous
- **Dinner:** Pan-seared tilapia with quinoa and sautéed green beans
- **Snack:** Fresh pear slices with a handful of pumpkin seeds

Day 9:

- **Breakfast:** Scrambled tofu with tomatoes, onions, and spinach
- **Lunch:** Turkey and vegetable stir-fry with brown rice
- **Dinner:** Grilled salmon with sweet potato fries and steamed broccoli
- **Snack:** Greek yogurt with a drizzle of honey

Day 10:

- **Breakfast:** Smoothie bowl with unsweetened almond milk, banana, and nuts/seeds mix
- **Lunch:** Lentil and vegetable wrap with whole-grain tortilla
- **Dinner:** Baked chicken thighs with quinoa and roasted Brussels sprouts
- **Snack:** Handful of almonds

Day 11:

- **Breakfast:** Cottage cheese and mango parfait
- **Lunch:** Quinoa and black bean burrito bowl with salsa and avocado
- **Dinner:** Grilled shrimp skewers with quinoa salad
- **Snack:** Apple slices with a tablespoon of almond butter

Day 12:

- **Breakfast:** Whole-grain oatmeal topped with sliced strawberries, chia seeds, and honey
- **Lunch:** Chickpea and vegetable stir-fry with brown rice
- **Dinner:** Baked cod with sweet potato mash and steamed asparagus
- **Snack:** Raw vegetables with hummus

Day 13:

- **Breakfast:** Protein smoothie with unsweetened almond milk, mixed berries, and protein powder
- **Lunch:** Egg salad lettuce wraps with cherry tomatoes
- **Dinner:** Lean beef and broccoli stir-fry with whole wheat noodles
- **Snack:** Cottage cheese with sliced peaches

Day 14:

- **Breakfast:** Avocado toast on whole-grain bread with poached eggs
- **Lunch:** Tuna salad with mixed greens, cucumbers, and whole-grain croutons
- **Dinner:** Baked chicken breast with quinoa and roasted cauliflower
- **Snack:** Handful of pistachios

Day 15:

- **Breakfast:** Whole-grain pancakes with fresh berries and Greek yogurt
- **Lunch:** Shredded chicken salad with mixed greens, cherry tomatoes, and vinaigrette
- **Dinner:** Grilled trout with lemon, quinoa, and sautéed asparagus
- **Snack:** Fresh pineapple chunks with a handful of mixed nuts

Day 16:

- **Breakfast:** Scrambled eggs with diced tomatoes, bell peppers, and whole-wheat toast
- **Lunch:** Turkey and avocado salad wrap with whole-grain tortilla
- **Dinner:** Baked salmon with sweet potato wedges and steamed green beans
- **Snack:** Greek yogurt with a sprinkle of granola

Day 17:

- **Breakfast:** Smoothie with unsweetened almond milk, banana, spinach, and protein powder
- **Lunch:** Lentil soup with whole-grain crackers
- **Dinner:** Stir-fried tofu with mixed vegetables and brown rice
- **Snack:** Handful of almonds

Day 18:

- **Breakfast:** Cottage cheese and berry smoothie bowl
- **Lunch:** Quinoa salad with black beans, corn, and diced tomatoes
- **Dinner:** Grilled chicken breast with quinoa and roasted Brussels sprouts
- **Snack:** Fresh apple slices with a tablespoon of almond butter

Day 19:

- **Breakfast:** Whole-grain oatmeal topped with sliced bananas, chia seeds, and honey
- **Lunch:** Chickpea and vegetable curry with brown rice
- **Dinner:** Grilled shrimp with quinoa salad and sautéed spinach
- **Snack:** Raw vegetables with hummus

Day 20:

- **Breakfast:** Protein smoothie with unsweetened almond milk, mixed berries, and chia seeds
- **Lunch:** Egg and vegetable stir-fry with brown rice
- **Dinner:** Lean beef stir-fry with broccoli and whole wheat noodles
- **Snack:** Cottage cheese with sliced peaches

Day 21:

- **Breakfast:** Avocado and poached egg on whole-grain toast
- **Lunch:** Tuna and quinoa salad with mixed greens and cherry tomatoes
- **Dinner:** Baked cod with quinoa and roasted cauliflower
- **Snack:** Handful of pistachios

Day 22:

- **Breakfast:** Whole-grain waffles with mixed berries and a dollop of Greek yogurt
- **Lunch:** Chicken and vegetable kebabs with whole-wheat couscous
- **Dinner:** Pan-seared tilapia with quinoa and sautéed green beans
- **Snack:** Fresh pear slices with a handful of pumpkin seeds

Day 23:

- **Breakfast:** Scrambled tofu with tomatoes, onions, and spinach
- **Lunch:** Turkey and vegetable stir-fry with brown rice
- **Dinner:** Grilled salmon with sweet potato fries and steamed broccoli
- **Snack:** Greek yogurt with a drizzle of honey

Day 24:

- **Breakfast:** Smoothie bowl with unsweetened almond milk, banana, and a mix of nuts and seeds
- **Lunch:** Lentil and vegetable wrap with whole-grain tortilla
- **Dinner:** Baked chicken thighs with quinoa and roasted Brussels sprouts
- **Snack:** Handful of almonds

Day 25:

- **Breakfast:** Cottage cheese and mango parfait
- **Lunch:** Quinoa and black bean burrito bowl with salsa and avocado
- **Dinner:** Grilled shrimp skewers with quinoa salad
- **Snack:** Apple slices with a tablespoon of almond butter

Day 26:

- **Breakfast:** Whole-grain oatmeal topped with sliced strawberries and chia seeds
- **Lunch:** Chickpea and vegetable stir-fry with brown rice
- **Dinner:** Baked cod with a side of sweet potato mash and steamed asparagus
- **Snack:** Raw vegetables with hummus

Day 27:

- **Breakfast:** Protein smoothie with unsweetened almond milk, mixed berries, and a scoop of protein powder
- **Lunch:** Egg salad lettuce wraps with cherry tomatoes
- **Dinner:** Lean beef and broccoli stir-fry with whole wheat noodles
- **Snack:** Cottage cheese with sliced peaches

Day 28:

- **Breakfast:** Avocado toast on whole-grain bread with poached eggs
- **Lunch:** Tuna salad with mixed greens, cucumbers, and whole-grain croutons
- **Dinner:** Baked chicken breast with quinoa and roasted cauliflower
- **Snack:** Handful of pistachios

Day 29:

- **Breakfast:** Whole-grain pancakes with fresh berries and a side of Greek yogurt
- **Lunch:** Shredded chicken salad with mixed greens, cherry tomatoes, and a light vinaigrette
- **Dinner:** Grilled trout with lemon, quinoa, and sautéed asparagus
- **Snack:** Fresh pineapple chunks with a handful of mixed nuts

Day 30:

- **Breakfast:** Scrambled eggs with diced tomatoes, bell peppers, and a slice of whole-wheat toast
- **Lunch:** Turkey and avocado salad wrap with whole-grain tortilla
- **Dinner:** Baked salmon with sweet potato wedges and steamed green beans

  Snack: Greek yogurt with a sprinkle of granola

Recipes

BREAKFAST RECIPES

Scrambled Veggie Breakfast Burrito

Ingredients:

- two huge eggs
- 1/4 cup bell peppers, chopped (any color)
- 1/4 cup chopped onions
- a quarter cup of chopped tomatoes
- 1/4 cup black beans, cooked
- 1 whole grain tortilla
- Season with salt and pepper to taste.
- Avocado slices (optional, for topping)
- Hot sauce or salsa (optional, for topping)

Instructions:

- Sauté the chopped bell peppers and onions in a nonstick pan until softened.
- In a bowl, whisk the eggs, then add them to the pan with the sautéed vegetables.
- Scramble the eggs and vegetables together until fully done.
- Combine the chopped tomatoes and cooked black beans in a mixing bowl.
- The whole wheat tortilla should be warmed.
- Fill the tortilla with the scrambled egg mixture.
- If desired, top with avocado slices.
- To make a burrito, roll up the tortilla.
- On the side, serve with salsa or spicy sauce.

Greek Yogurt Parfait

Ingredients:

- 1 cup plain Greek yogurt (plain, unsweetened)
- 1/2 cup berries, mixed (blueberries, strawberries, raspberries)
- 2 tbsp. nuts, chopped (almonds, walnuts, or mixed)
- 1 tbsp honey (or maple syrup)
- 1 teaspoon chia seeds

Instructions:

- In a glass or bowl, layer half of the Greek yogurt.
- Add a layer of mixed berries on top of the yogurt.
- Sprinkle half of the chopped nuts and chia seeds over the berries.
- Drizzle half of the honey or maple syrup over the layers.
- Repeat the layers with the remaining ingredients.
- Enjoy the parfait with a spoon.

Veggie Omelets with Spinach and Feta

Ingredients:

- three huge eggs
- 1/4 cup spinach, chopped
- 2 tbsp. crumbled feta cheese
- a quarter cup of chopped tomatoes
- Season with salt and pepper to taste.
  Cooking spray or olive oil

Instructions:

- Prepare a pan that does not stick by heating it over medium heat and adding a tiny quantity of cooking spray or olive oil (optional).
- Beat the eggs in a bowl until they are completely incorporated.

- Pour the eggs that have been whisked into the skillet.

- While the eggs are beginning to set, sprinkle the sliced tomatoes, crumbled feta cheese, and chopped spinach over one side of the omelet.

- Use pepper and salt to season the food.

- Before gently folding the remaining half of the omelet over the filling, wait until the eggs have reached the desired level of doneness but are still somewhat runny on top.

- The omelet should be cooked for one more minute until it is completely set.

- Take the omelet and place it on a platter before serving.

Berry Protein Smoothie Bowl

Ingredients:

- 1 cup berries, mixed (blueberries, strawberries, raspberries)

- 1 frozen banana

- 1/2 cup plain Greek yogurt (plain, unsweetened)

- 1 protein powder scoop (vanilla or berry-flavored)

- a quarter cup of almond milk (or any preferred milk)

  Toppings: sliced almonds, chia seeds, and strawberries, sliced

Instructions:

- Put the frozen bananas, Greek yogurt, protein powder, and almond milk into a blender. Blend until smooth. Mix in the mixed berries.
- Puree till it is silky smooth and creamy. To obtain the correct consistency, you may need to add more almond milk.
- The smoothie should be poured into a bowl.
- Almonds, chia seeds, and strawberries cut into slices should be sprinkled over top.
- Utilize a spoon to enjoy.

Avocado and Egg Breakfast Toast

Ingredients:

- 1 piece toasted whole grain bread
- 1/2 ripe avocado, mashed
- 1 poached or fried egg
- Season with salt and pepper to taste
- Red pepper flakes (optional, for extra flavor)
- Chopped cilantro or parsley (for garnish)

Instructions:

- The whole grain bread should be toasted.
- Distribute the mashed avocado equally on top of the toasted bread.
- Serve with a poached or fried egg on top.

- If desired, season with salt, pepper, and red pepper flakes.

- Garnish with cilantro or parsley, if desired.

- Serve the avocado and egg toast right away.

Nutty Banana Chia Pudding

Ingredients:

- 2 tbsp of chia seeds

- a half-cup of almond milk (or any preferred milk)

- 1 mashed ripe banana

- 1 tablespoon nuts, chopped (walnuts, almonds, or mixed)

- 1 tbsp honey (or maple syrup)

- a half teaspoon of vanilla extract

- a pinch of cinnamon

Instructions:

- Chia seeds and almond milk should be combined in a bowl. Stir well and set aside for a few minutes to thicken.

- Combine the mashed banana, chopped almonds, honey or maple syrup, vanilla essence, and cinnamon in a mixing bowl.

- Refrigerate the bowl overnight or for at least a few hours.

- Give the chia pudding a quick swirl before serving to mix all of the ingredients.

- As a creamy and healthy breakfast, serve the nutty banana chia pudding.

LUNCH RECIPES

Grilled Chicken and Quinoa Salad

Ingredients:

- 4 ounces sliced grilled chicken breast
- 1 cup quinoa, cooked
- 2 cups greens, mixed
- 1/2 cup halved cherry tomatoes
- 1/4 cup cucumber slices
- 1/4 cup red onion, chopped
- 1/4 cup feta cheese, crumbled
- Vinaigrette with balsamic vinegar (homemade or store-bought)

Instructions:

- Combine mixed greens, cherry tomatoes, sliced cucumbers, and chopped red onion in a large mixing dish.
- Top with the cooked quinoa and sliced grilled chicken.
- Toss gently with the balsamic vinaigrette to mix.
- Sprinkle the salad with crumbled feta cheese.
- As a filling and nutrient-dense lunch, serve the grilled chicken and quinoa salad.

Veggie and Hummus Wrap

Ingredients:

- 1 whole grain tortilla

- a quarter cup of hummus (any flavor)

- 1 cup of mixed greens

- 1/4 cup carrots, shredded

- 1/4 cup bell peppers, sliced

- 1/4 cup cucumber, sliced

- 2 tbsp. crumbled feta cheese (optional)

- Season with salt and pepper to taste.

Instructions:

- Place the whole wheat tortilla on a clean surface and flatten it.

- Spread hummus evenly on the tortilla.

- On top of the hummus, layer mixed greens, shredded carrots, sliced bell peppers, and sliced cucumber.

- If using, top with crumbled feta cheese.

- Season to taste with salt and pepper.

- To make a wrap, roll the tortilla firmly.

- Serve by cutting the wrap in half diagonally.

Lentil and Vegetable Stir-Fry

Ingredients:

- 1 cup green lentils, cooked
- 1 cup chopped veggies (bell peppers, snap peas, carrots, broccoli)
- 2 minced garlic cloves
- 1 tablespoon soy sauce (low sodium)
- 1 tbsp sesame oil
- 1/2 teaspoon minced ginger
- 1/4 teaspoon crushed red pepper flakes (adjust to taste)
- Green onions, chopped, for garnish

Instructions:

- Heat sesame oil in a large pan or wok over medium-high heat.
- Sauté the minced garlic and ginger for approximately 30 seconds, or until fragrant.
- Stir in the mixed veggies for a few minutes, or until slightly tender.
- Incorporate the cooked green lentils.
- Toss the stir-fry with low-sodium soy sauce to mix.
- To add a little spice, sprinkle with red pepper flakes.
- Cook for another 1-3 minutes, stirring often.
- Before serving, garnish with chopped green onions.

Quinoa and Black Bean Bowl

Ingredients:

- 1 cup quinoa, cooked
- 1/2 cup washed and drained black beans
- 1/2 cup bell peppers, diced (any color)
- 1/4 cup red onion, chopped
- 1/4 cup kernels of corn (fresh, frozen, or canned)
- 2 tbsp fresh cilantro, chopped
- One lime juice
- Season with salt and pepper to taste.
- Avocado slices (optional, for topping)
- Sour cream or Greek yogurt (optional, for topping)

Instructions:

- Combine cooked quinoa, black beans, diced bell peppers, diced red onion, and corn kernels in a mixing dish.
- Squeeze lime juice over the mixture and add chopped cilantro.
- Toss everything together until everything is fully integrated.
- Season to taste with salt and pepper.
- Serve in bowls, topped with sliced avocado and, if wanted, a dollop of Greek yogurt or sour cream.

Mediterranean Chickpea Salad

Ingredients:

- 1 can (15 oz) washed and drained chickpeas

- 1 cup cucumber, diced

- 1 cup halved cherry tomatoes

- 1/2 cup red onion, chopped

- 1/4 cup feta cheese, crumbled

- 1/4 cup pitted and sliced Kalamata olives

- 2 tbsp fresh parsley, chopped

- 1 lemon juice

- 2 tbsp extra virgin olive oil

- Season with salt and pepper to taste.

Instructions:

- Chickpeas, diced cucumber, cherry tomatoes, diced red onion, crumbled feta cheese, and sliced Kalamata olives should be mixed in a big bowl.

- The salad should be topped with chopped parsley, lemon juice, and extra-virgin olive oil, depending on your preference.

- The components should be carefully mixed by tossing.

- Add salt and pepper to taste, and season with salt.

- As a lunch option that is both reviving and nourishing, serve the chickpea salad from the Mediterranean.

Turkey and Avocado Lettuce Wraps

Ingredients:

- 4 hefty lettuce leaves (such as romaine or butter lettuce)
- 4 ounces cooked and sliced lean turkey breast
- 1/2 sliced avocado
- 1/4 cup carrots, shredded
- 1/4 cup bell peppers, chopped (any color)
- hummus (two tablespoons) (any flavor)
- Garnish with fresh cilantro leaves

Instructions:

- Place the lettuce leaves on a clean surface, flat.
- On each lettuce leaf, spread a thin coating of hummus.
- On top of the hummus, layer sliced turkey breast, avocado slices, shredded carrots, and chopped bell peppers.
- Garnish with fresh cilantro leaves if desired.
- Wrap the lettuce leaves firmly together.
- If necessary, secure with toothpicks and serve.

Roasted Veggie and Quinoa Bowl

Ingredients:

- 1 cup quinoa, cooked
- 1 cup roasted mixed veggies (bell peppers, zucchini, eggplant, etc.)
- 1/4 cup crumbled feta or goat cheese
- 2 tbsp fresh basil, chopped
- 1 tbsp. balsamic vinegar
- 1 tbsp olive oil (extra virgin)
- Season with salt and pepper to taste.

Instructions:

- Combine cooked quinoa and roasted veggies in a mixing dish.
- To the mixture, add crumbled goat cheese or feta cheese and chopped basil.
- Drizzle the bowl with balsamic vinegar and extra-virgin olive oil.
- Season to taste with salt and pepper.
- Toss everything together until everything is fully integrated.
- As a filling and savory lunch, serve the roasted vegetable and quinoa dish.

DINNER RECIPES

Grilled Salmon with Quinoa and Steamed Vegetables

Ingredients:

- 1 fillet of salmon

- 1 cooked cup of quinoa

- Steamed mixed veggies (broccoli, carrots, asparagus, etc.)

- Garnish with lemon wedges

- Extra virgin olive oil

- Herbs, fresh (such as dill or parsley)

- Season with salt and pepper to taste.

Instructions:

- First, bring the grill or grill pan up to a temperature of medium-high.

- Salt and pepper should be applied to the salmon fillet after it has been brushed with olive oil.

- Cook the salmon on the grill for about four to five minutes on each side, or until it can be easily flaked with a fork.

- While the salmon is cooking on the grill, prepare the quinoa according to the directions provided on the box.

- Steam the veggies in a mixture until they are soft.

- Place the grilled salmon on a platter, and accompany it with quinoa that has been prepared and veggies that have been steamed.

- It is recommended to drizzle the salmon with a little amount of olive oil, squeeze lemon juice over it, and garnish it with fresh herbs.
- Experience a supper that is both nourishing and delicious.

Turkey and Veggie Stir-Fry

Ingredients:

- 4 ounces lean ground turkey
- 1 cup stir-fry veggies (bell peppers, snap peas, carrots, broccoli, etc.)
- 2 garlic cloves, minced
- 1 tbsp low-sodium soy sauce
- 1/2 tsp sesame oil
- 1 teaspoon minced ginger
- Red pepper flakes (adjust to taste)
- Green onions, chopped
- cooked brown rice or quinoa

Instructions:

- Heat sesame oil in a large pan or wok over medium-high heat.
- Sauté the minced garlic and ginger for approximately 30 seconds, or until fragrant.
- Cook until the lean ground turkey is browned and cooked thoroughly.

- Stir-fry the mixed stir-fry veggies for a few minutes, or until slightly soft.

- Toss the stir-fry with low-sodium soy sauce to mix.

- Red pepper flakes may be used for more flavor and spiciness.

- Serve the turkey and vegetable stir-fry with brown rice or quinoa.

- Before serving, garnish with chopped green onions.

Baked Chicken with Roasted Vegetables

Ingredients:

- 2 skinless, boneless chicken breasts

- 2 cups roasted mixed veggies (sweet potatoes, bell peppers, zucchini, etc.)

- 2 tbsp of olive oil

- 1 tsp. dry herbs (such as thyme, rosemary, or oregano)

- Season with salt and pepper to taste.

Instructions:

- Preheat the oven to 400 degrees Fahrenheit (200 degrees Celsius).

- Olive oil, dried herbs, salt, and pepper should be incorporated with the roasted veggies that have been mixed.

- Prepare a baking sheet that has been lined with parchment paper and place the chicken breasts on it.

- Salt and pepper the chicken breasts, and then spray them with olive oil. Season with salt and pepper.

- On the baking sheet, arrange the veggies that have been seasoned in a circle around the chicken breasts.

- Bake for about twenty to twenty-five minutes in an oven that has been preheated, or until the chicken is completely cooked through and the veggies are soft.

- After removing the chicken from the oven, let it rest for a few minutes before slicing it.

- To create a supper that is both healthful and delectable, serve the baked chicken with veggies that have been roasted.

Lentil and Vegetable Stuffed Bell Peppers

Ingredients:

- 3 medium bell peppers (any color)

- 1 cup green lentils, cooked

- 1 pound chopped tomatoes

- 1/2 cup zucchini, diced

- 1/4 cup red onion, chopped

- 1/4 cup shredded mozzarella (or other preferred cheese)

- 2 minced garlic cloves

- 1 teaspoon Italian dried herbs (oregano, basil, thyme)

- Season with salt and pepper to taste.

- Extra virgin olive oil

- Garnish with fresh parsley

Instructions:

- Preheat the oven to 375 degrees Fahrenheit (190 degrees Celsius).

- Remove the tops of the bell peppers and the seeds and membranes.

- Warm the olive oil in a pan over medium heat. Cook until the minced garlic, diced zucchini, chopped red onion, and dried Italian herbs are softened.

- Cooked green lentils and chopped tomatoes should be added now. Season with salt and pepper to taste.

- Fill the bell peppers halfway with the lentil-vegetable mixture.

- In a baking dish, place the filled bell peppers.

- Top each bell pepper with shredded mozzarella or your favorite cheese.

- Cover the baking dish with aluminum foil and bake for 25-30 minutes, or until the peppers are soft and the cheese has melted.

- Before serving, garnish with fresh parsley.

Teriyaki Tofu Stir-Fry

Ingredients:

- 8 ounces cubed firm tofu 2 cups mixed stir-fry veggies (bell peppers, snap peas, carrots, broccoli, etc.)
- 2 tbsp teriyaki sauce (low sodium)
- 1 tbsp sesame seed oil
- 1 teaspoon of soy sauce (low-sodium)
- 1/2 teaspoon ginger, minced
- 1 minced garlic clove
- Brown rice or quinoa, cooked

Instructions:

- After pressing the tofu to remove any extra water, cut it into cubes.
- To prepare the marinade, put the following ingredients in a bowl: teriyaki sauce, sesame oil, soy sauce, minced ginger, and minced garlic.
- Tofu cubes should be marinated in the marinade for about fifteen to twenty minutes.
- A small amount of sesame oil should be heated slightly over medium-high heat in a big pan or wok.
- The tofu that has been marinated should be stir-fried until it is golden brown and slightly crunchy.

- After a few minutes, add the mixed stir-fry veggies and continue to stir-fry them until they are cooked.

- Spread a tiny bit of more teriyaki sauce over the stir-fry, and then toss it to coat everything.

- The teriyaki tofu stir-fry should be served over quinoa or brown rice that has been prepared.

Mediterranean Grilled Veggie Wrap

Ingredients:

- 1 tortilla (whole wheat)

- 1 tablespoon hummus (any flavor)

- Vegetables grilled or roasted (bell peppers, zucchini, eggplant, red onion)

- pitted and sliced Kalamata olives

- Feta crumbled

- basil leaves

- season with salt and pepper to taste

Instructions:

- Place the whole wheat tortilla on a clean surface and flatten it.

- Spread hummus on top of the tortilla.

- On top of the hummus, layer grilled or roasted veggies.

- Combine sliced Kalamata olives, crumbled feta cheese, and fresh basil leaves in a mixing bowl.

- Season to taste with salt and pepper.
- To make a wrap, roll the tortilla firmly.
- Serve by cutting the wrap in half diagonally.

Managing Cravings and Detox Symptoms

When adopting a dietary alteration, such as the Metabolic Confusion Diet for endomorphs, managing cravings and possible detox symptoms is crucial to your overall performance and well-being. Here are some tips to help you deal with these difficulties:

- **Keep Hydrated:** Cravings and dehydration may sometimes be mistaken. Drinking enough water throughout the day may help to reduce the intensity of cravings.
- **Balanced Meals:** Include lean protein, healthy fats, and fiber-rich carbohydrates in your meals. This may help with blood sugar regulation and desire decrease.
- **Include Fiber:** Fiber-rich foods like vegetables, fruits, and whole grains help keep you feeling full and satisfied, reducing your chances of cravings.
- **Consumption of Protein:** Protein-rich meals may help regulate hunger and cravings. To stay satiated, include lean protein sources in each meal.
- **Choose healthful snacks** such as nuts, seeds, Greek yogurt, and fruits if you experience between-meal cravings.

- **Gradual Transition:** If you're making big dietary changes, attempt to do it gradually. Increased desires and discomfort may come from abrupt and drastic changes.

- **Mindful Eating:** Be mindful of symptoms of hunger and fullness. Eat slowly and carefully to prevent overeating and undesired urges.

- **Healthy Fats:** Include healthy fats in your diet such as avocados, almonds, and olive oil. They may help with hunger and satiety.

- **Plan ahead of time your meals and snacks**. Having healthy alternatives on hand may help you avoid making poor choices.

- **Allow Occasional Treats:** Deprivation may lead to strong urges. Allow yourself periodic indulgences in moderation to satisfy cravings and remain on track.

- **Stress Management:** Cravings may be triggered by stress. Incorporate stress-relieving hobbies such as meditation, yoga, or deep breathing into your daily routine.

- **Get Enough Sleep:** Sleep deprivation may increase cravings, especially for sugary foods. Aim for 7-9 hours of quality sleep each night.

- **Mindset Shift:** Focus on the benefits of your dietary choices, such as more energy, better health, and accomplishing your objectives. This upbeat mindset may help you regulate your desires.

Detoxification Symptoms:

If you experience detox symptoms such as headaches, tiredness, or irritability when transitioning to a new diet, here are some strategies to help manage them:

- ***Gradual Transition:*** If you're experiencing severe detox symptoms, it might be due to a rapid transition. Reduce your use of processed foods, sugar, and caffeine gradually rather than suddenly.

- ***Hydration:*** Drinking water may help remove toxins and alleviate certain detox symptoms.

- **Herbal teas,** such as ginger, chamomile, and peppermint, might assist in relaxing the body during detox.

- **Rest and sleep:** Allow your body to rest and mend throughout the detox phase. Adequate sleep may help your body repair.

- **Gentle activity,** such as walking, stretching, or yoga, might help improve circulation and reduce discomfort.

- **Nutrient-Dense Foods:** To aid your body's natural detoxification processes, consume nutrient-dense meals such as leafy greens, cruciferous vegetables, and antioxidants.

Macronutrient Cycling Phase 2

Understanding the Different Macronutrients

Understanding the different macronutrients is crucial for developing a balanced and effective nutritional plan, such as the Metabolic Confusion Diet for endomorphs. Macronutrients are essential nutrients that provide energy to the body and are required in large amounts. The three primary macronutrients are carbohydrates, proteins, and lipids. Here's a summary of each:

Carbohydrates: *Carbohydrates are the body's primary source of energy. They are broken down into glucose, which is utilized to power many bodily activities, including brain function and physical activity. There are two kinds of carbohydrates:*

- Simple Carbohydrates are sugars found in foods like fruits, honey, and milk. While they provide instant energy, they may cause blood sugar spikes and crashes.

Complex Carbs: Due to their delayed digestion and fiber content, complex carbohydrates found in foods such as whole grains (oats, quinoa, brown rice), vegetables, legumes, and starchy meals provide prolonged energy.

Proteins: *Proteins are necessary for tissue creation and repair, enzyme and hormone synthesis, and immune system maintenance.*

Proteins are built up of amino acids, which are regarded as the body's "building blocks." Dietary protein sources include:

- Animal proteins include lean meats, poultry, fish, eggs, and dairy products.
- Plant protein is abundant in beans, lentils, nuts, seeds, tofu, tempeh, and certain grains (quinoa, amaranth).
- Protein amino acids are classified as either essential (obtained from food) or non-essential (obtained through supplementation) (made by the organism). To receive all of the necessary amino acids, it is vital to eat a variety of protein sources.

Fats: *Fats are necessary for several bodily activities, including hormone production, nutrition absorption, insulation, and energy storage. Fats come in a variety of forms:*

- Saturated fats, which are present in animal products (meat and dairy), as well as certain tropical oils, should be consumed in moderation since excessive intake may raise cholesterol levels.
- Monounsaturated fats are heart-healthy fats found in olive oil, avocados, and almonds.
- Omega-3 and omega-6 fatty acids are examples of polyunsaturated fats. Fatty fish (salmon, mackerel), flaxseeds, walnuts, and some oils are all high in omega-3 fatty acids.

Trans Fats: These fats, which are created artificially by hydrogenation, are found in certain processed foods and should be avoided since they may raise dangerous cholesterol levels.

The Metabolic Confusion Diet promotes proper macronutrient balance to improve metabolism, energy levels, and weight control. Each macronutrient is essential for good health; the trick is to emphasize high-quality sources:

Carbohydrates: Select complex carbohydrate sources including whole grains, vegetables, and legumes. Reduce your consumption of added sugars and processed carbohydrates.

Proteins: Include lean protein sources, both animal and plant-based, in your diet. Vary your protein sources to get a diverse amino acid composition.

Healthy fats should be emphasized, such as those found in nuts, seeds, avocados, and fatty fish. Reduce your consumption of saturated and trans fats.

Endomorph Cycling Patterns Development

Designing optimal cycle patterns for endomorphs in the context of the Metabolic Confusion Diet includes devising a systematic strategy that alternates macronutrient ratios, calorie intake, and meal timing. The goal is to increase metabolism, promote fat loss, and retain muscle mass. Endomorph cycling patterns may be created in the following ways:

Macronutrient Cycling: On various days of the week, vary the macronutrient distribution (carbohydrates, proteins, and fats). This may help with fat loss by reducing metabolic adaptation.

- On active or exercise days, carbohydrate intake should be increased. Focus on complex carbs such as whole grains, fruits, and vegetables to fuel energy needs and recovery.
- On days of rest or low-intensity activity, maintain a moderate carbohydrate intake. This gives you energy without consuming too many calories.
- Low-Carb Days: Schedule low-carb days regularly to encourage the body to burn stored fat for energy. This may help you break past plateaus.

Calorie Cycling: Calorie cycling is the technique of alternating calorie intake to prevent the body from adapting to a regular diet. This is particularly beneficial for endomorphs who may experience fat loss plateaus.

- Increase calorie consumption before and after exercises or on more active days to support energy needs and recovery.
- Low-Calorie Days: To create a calorie deficit, lower calorie intake on rest days or days with low activity levels.

Intermittent Fasting: This involves alternating between eating and fasting times. This may help endomorphs control their calorie intake and improve their insulin sensitivity.

- Using the 16/8 approach, fast for 16 hours and eat within an 8-hour window. This is particularly good for persons who eat bigger meals regularly.
- The 12/12 Method is a softer variant of fasting that involves fasting for 12 hours and eating within 12 hours.

Adjust meal times according to exercise level and nutritional needs.

- Pre-Exercise Nutrition: Consume a balanced breakfast or snack including carbs and protein 1-2 hours before your workout to provide energy and help in muscle regeneration.
- Post-Exercise Nutrition: To assist recovery, have a high-protein, high-carbohydrate meal within an hour following an intensive workout.
- Include re-feed days when carbohydrate intake is purposefully increased. This may help replace glycogen stores, boost metabolism, and provide mental relaxation after dieting.

Pay Attention to Your Body: Be aware of your appetite, energy levels, and how your body responds to different cycle patterns. Make necessary changes to the approach to ensure its long-term sustainability and effectiveness.

Optimizing Nutrient Timing for Energy Balance

Optimizing meal timing is crucial for achieving energy balance and achieving your goals, whether they be weight loss, muscle growth, or overall health. Nutrient timing is the purposeful act of selecting when to consume certain nutrients (carbohydrates, proteins, and fats) to maximize their benefits. Here are some pointers to help you optimize your diet timing for energy balance:

Nutrition Before Exercise:

The idea is to optimize performance by fueling your workout.

Strategies:

- Consume a well-balanced meal. 1-2 hours before working out.
- For long-term energy, prioritize complex carbohydrates (healthy grains, fruits, and vegetables).
- Include a little amount of lean protein for muscle support.
- Maintain a modest fat intake to avoid stomach pain when exercising.

Post-Workout Nutrition:

The goal is to help with recovery, muscle regeneration, and glycogen replacement.

Strategies:

- Consume a meal or snack within an hour after concluding your exercise.

- Consume a mix of carbohydrates and protein to replenish glycogen and aid muscle repair.

- Use easily digestible proteins for rapid absorption (whey, lean meats, plant-based sources).

- Provide healthy fats for overall nutritional balance.

Well-balanced meals:

The objective is to keep energy levels consistent and provide essential nutrients throughout the day.

Strategies:

- Aim for well-balanced meals, with a range of carbohydrates, proteins, and healthy fats.

- Choose complex carbs and fiber-rich meals to slow digestion and provide long-lasting energy.

- Include lean proteins to assist your muscles in maintaining and repairing.

- Increase satiety and nutrient absorption by including healthy fats.

Snacks:

The idea is to minimize energy dips between meals while also controlling appetite.

- Snack on nutrient-dense meals that include carbs and protein.
- A small handful of nuts, a piece of fruit with Greek yogurt, or carrot sticks with hummus are all options.
- Avoid high-sugar or high-fat snacks, which may trigger energy slumps.

Nighttime nutrition:

The goal is to help in recovery and to manage nighttime fasting.

- Dinner should consist of lean protein, healthy fats, and non-starchy vegetables.
- Limit high carbohydrates before bedtime to minimize sleep disruptions.
- Large meals before bedtime should be avoided since they might interfere with digestion and sleep quality.

Hydration is critical.

The objective is to maintain enough hydration for optimum energy levels and physical functions.

- Drink water throughout the day and adjust your intake depending on your activity level and the weather.
- Hydrate before, during, and after physical exercise to avoid dehydration.
- Choose water as your main beverage and limit your intake of sugary drinks and coffee.

Be Mindful of Your Body:

Strategies:

- Pay attention to hunger and fullness indications to help you plan your meals.
- Portion sizes should be changed depending on your degree of activity and your objectives.
- Individualize nutrition timing depending on your preferences and needs.

Phase 3: Movement and Exercise Strategies

Developing Endomorph Workouts

Endomorph exercises need a fitness regimen that takes their body type, talents, and difficulties into account. Endomorphs have a higher body fat percentage and may find it easier to gain weight, but with the right strategy, they may achieve their fitness goals. Endomorph training should be adjusted in the following ways:

Cardiovascular exercise is important since it burns calories and aids in weight reduction. Use both moderate-intensity and high-intensity interval training (HIIT) sessions to increase calorie expenditure.

Strength training is important for growing lean muscle mass, which may help with metabolism and body composition. Compound training involving many muscle groups should be prioritized:

- Lunges, Squats, and Deadlifts
- Bench press workouts
- Rows and overhead presses

Circuit training is a fast-paced strategy that combines aerobic and strength exercises. This may help you burn more calories while also improving your cardiovascular fitness and muscular growth.

Progressive Overload: Gradually increase the weight or resistance you lift over time. This increases muscle growth and keeps plateaus at bay.

High-Intensity Interval Training (HIIT) involves alternating between quick bursts of intense exercise and brief periods of rest. It stimulates metabolism, burns calories and enhances cardiovascular fitness.

Endomorphs depend greatly on consistency and frequency. To maintain momentum and produce results, strive for at least 3-5 times a week of exercise.

Nutrition: A well-balanced diet rich in nutrient-dense meals should be supplemented with your exercises. This may boost energy levels, recovery time, and overall wellness.

Sleep and Recuperation: Prioritize sleep and recovery. Because muscles renew and grow during rest, obtaining adequate sleep is essential for success.

Mindful Eating: Keep track of your meal portions and prevent overeating. Mindful eating may assist you in avoiding consuming too many calories.

Variability: Vary your workouts to prevent adaptation and maintain your drive. This entails changing the intensity and pattern of training.

Full-Body Exercises: Include full-body workouts that target many muscle groups in each session. This may assist you in burning more calories and building more muscle.

Advice from an expert: Speak with a personal trainer or fitness consultant who is knowledgeable about endomorph body types. They may design a personalized fitness program and provide advice on proper form and development.

Patience is required, particularly for endomorphs who wish to decrease weight. Be patient and focus on taking modest moves ahead.

Combining strength and cardiovascular exercise is recommended.

Incorporating strength training and aerobic exercise into your fitness routine may provide a well-rounded approach to improving fitness, muscle development, and overall health. Here's how to efficiently include both types of workout:

1. ***Plan Your Workouts for the Week:*** Make a plan for your week's workouts, designating certain days for strength training and aerobic activities. This fosters consistency and prevents overtraining.

2. ***Determine Your Priorities:*** Determine if your primary goal is muscle building, fat reduction, or overall fitness. Adjust the strength-to-cardio ratio according to your objectives.

3. ***Mix cardio and strength training:*** Set aside certain days for each kind of workout. For example, strength training on Mondays, Wednesdays, and Fridays, and aerobics on Tuesdays and Thursdays.

Same Session: You may also combine the two types of workouts in the same session. Begin with strength training and work your way up to cardio (or vice versa). This strategy may help you save time while burning more calories.

4. ***Warm-Up and Cool-Down:*** Regardless of method, always begin with an active warm-up to prepare your muscles for exercise and reduce the risk of injury. Finish with a cool-down and static stretches to aid in healing.

5. ***Modify Intensity:*** Include a mix of moderate-intensity steady-state cardio (e.g., brisk walking, jogging) and high-intensity interval training (HIIT). HIIT may be more efficient and effective in terms of calorie burn.

Strength Training Intensity: Focus on progressive overload by gradually increasing the weight or resistance utilized in strength training. This promotes muscle growth and strength.

6. ***Recovery Days:*** Include rest or active recovery days to minimize overtraining. These days, gentle activities such as yoga, stretching, or mild walking may be added.

7. ***Progression and Adaptation:*** Adjust your training regimen frequently to prevent plateaus. Increase weights, change

routines, and reduce aerobic intensity as your fitness level improves.

New Weekly Workout Split

Day One Strength Training

- Priority should be given to compound exercises (squats, deadlifts, and bench presses).
- Each exercise takes three to four sets of eight to twelve repetitions.

Day 2 Cardiovascular Exercise

- Select an activity that you like (for example, jogging, cycling, or swimming).
- It is advised that you do 30-45 minutes of moderate-intensity aerobics.

Day 3 Strength Training

- Include a range of exercises that target various muscle groups.
- Use heavier weights for fewer repetitions (3-5 sets of 5-8 reps).

Day 4: Cardio and Core Workout

- Core exercises should be performed after a 20-minute HIIT session.

- 30 seconds of high-intensity exercise (such as sprinting) followed by 30 seconds of rest, for example. Repeat for a total of 20 minutes.

Day 5: Rest or Active Recovery?

Day 6: Full-Body Strength Training

- Compound and isolation training should be combined.
- 3 to 4 sets of 8 to 12 repetitions.

Day 7: Cardio and flexibility training

- Opt for a low-impact aerobic exercise (for example, walking or cycling).
- Finish with a stretching or yoga session.

Finding the Right Mix of Intensity and Recovery

Finding the right balance of effort and recovery is crucial for optimizing fitness gains, preventing burnout, and improving overall health. Successfully balancing the two ensures that you are pushing your body while also enabling it to heal and thrive. Here's how to find a happy medium:

- Pay Attention to Your Body: Pay attention to how you feel during and after exercises. If you're always fatigued, sore, or mentally drained, it might be a sign that you need more rest.

- **Alternate Intensity:** Alternate between high- and moderate-intensity exercises. Intense exercises put your body to the test, whilst moderate programs promote active recovery.

- **Progressive Overload:** Gradually increase the intensity of your exercises over time. This might indicate lifting more weights, sprinting faster, or performing more challenging routines.

- **Active Recovery Days:** Include active recovery days in your routine. Walking, swimming, and light yoga are all activities that may help increase circulation and muscle recovery.

- **Include Rest Days:** It is vital to include regular rest days in your calendar. You should avoid or limit physical exertion on these days to allow your body to completely recover.

- Make enough sleep a priority since it is critical for recovery and overall health. Aim for 7-9 hours of sleep every night.

- **Nutrition:** A nutrient-dense, well-balanced diet may aid in recovery. Protein intake is critical for muscle repair and growth.

- **Stretching and foam rolling:** Incorporate foam rolling and stretching into your routine to reduce muscle tension and promote flexibility.

- Keep a workout journal to keep track of how you're feeling, how you're doing, and any changes in your body. This enables you to see trends and adjust your approach appropriately.

- Recognize Pain Indications: Distinguish between muscle discomfort and pain. While some stiffness is normal after exercise, prolonged pain or discomfort should not be ignored.

- Try ice baths, contrast baths (alternating hot and cold water), and massage to help reduce muscle soreness and speed healing.

- Individualization: Keep in mind that everyone's recovery needs are different. Age, fitness level, and heredity may all influence how much rest you need.

- Include high-intensity intervals followed by low-intensity phases in your periodization. This may aid in avoiding burnout and hastening long-term progress.

- Stress, Fatigue, and Emotional Well-Being: Address stress, fatigue, and emotional well-being. Engage in activities that are calming and unwinding.

- Seek expert help: Speak with a fitness consultant or a personal trainer. They may be able to help you in establishing a well-structured program that balances intensity and recuperation based on your aims and circumstances.

Managing Obstacles and Deadlines

Taking Care of Emotional Eating and Mental Blocks

Dealing with emotional eating and mental blocks is essential for having a positive relationship with food, accomplishing physical goals, and maintaining overall well-being. Here are some strategies for overcoming mental blockages and coping with emotional eating:

- Recognize Triggers: Recognize what triggers your emotional eating. Common reasons include stress, boredom, depression, loneliness, and worry.

- Mindful Eating means paying full attention to the sensory experience of eating without judgment. It might help you distinguish between physical hunger and emotional symptoms.

- Keep a food journal: Keep a food journal to track your meals and emotions to find patterns of emotional eating. This may help you become more aware of your eating habits.

- Develop Healthy Coping Strategies: Consider alternatives to using food to cope with emotions. Exercise, writing, meditating, and spending time with family and friends are all examples of pleasurable hobbies.

- Create a Routine: Schedule regular meal times to prevent being too hungry, which may lead to impulsive and emotional eating.

- Take a Minute to Pause Before Eating: When you sense the want to eat, take a minute to pause. Consider if you are hungry or if there is an emotional trigger at work.

- Develop Self-Compassion: Be kind to yourself and refrain from self-criticism. Recognize that emotional eating is a frequent issue and that it is OK to seek therapy and make positive changes.

- Address Emotional Needs: Seek professional treatment, such as therapy or counseling, to address underlying emotional difficulties that contribute to emotional eating.

- Visualize Your Objectives: Draw a mental image of your fitness and health goals. When confronted with emotional triggers, this may assist you in making better judgments.

- Use Positive Affirmations to Combat Negative Thoughts and Beliefs: Use positive affirmations to combat negative thoughts and beliefs that may be causing emotional eating.

- Reach out to friends, family, or support groups who share your fitness and health objectives. A robust support network may have a significant influence.

- Set realistic expectations: Avoid too strict restrictions or demands. Allow yourself to enjoy pleasures in moderation while keeping long-term objectives in mind.

- Consult a Licensed Dietitian, therapist, or counselor who specializes in emotional eating and behavior management if emotional eating is firmly ingrained or causes pain.

- Deal with Perfectionism: Perfectionism may lead to an all-or-nothing mindset. Accept progress over perfection and celebrate little victories.

- Create a thanksgiving practice to refocus your attention away from bad feelings and toward the great aspects of your life.

- Techniques for Visualization: Visualize yourself overcoming emotional eating issues and creating a healthy relationship with food.

- Reward Yourself for Non-Food Accomplishments: Reward yourself for non-food achievements such as meeting fitness goals, learning a new skill, or practicing self-care.

Overcoming Weight Loss Stagnation

Breaking through weight loss plateaus may be challenging, but with purposeful modifications to your diet, exercise program, and mindset, you can overcome them and keep progressing toward your goals. Here are a few effective methods for breaking through a weight loss plateau:

- Rethink Your Calorie Intake: As you lose weight, your body's calorie needs may change. To create a calorie deficit, recalculate your daily calorie requirements and adjust your intake accordingly.

- Intermittent fasting: By altering your eating patterns, intermittent fasting may help accelerate weight loss.

Experiment with different fasting windows to see if you can break through the plateau.

- Alter Your Training Routine: Vary your workout routine to keep your body guessing and minimize adaptation. Introduce new exercises, raise the intensity, or try a new style of cardio or strength training.

- Increase Intensity: Push yourself harder throughout workouts. Increase your weight, the duration of your workouts, or the intensity of your cardio sessions.

- High-intensity interval exercise will increase your calorie burn and metabolic rate (HIIT). HIIT exercises should be done a couple of times a week to aid in fat loss.

- Change Macronutrient Ratios: Experiment with adjusting your macronutrient ratios, such as increasing protein intake while slightly lowering carbohydrates. Protein may aid in feeling full and maintaining muscle mass.

- Recalculate Portion Sizes: Portion sizes may gradually increase over time. Rethink your meal sizes to prevent unintentionally consuming more calories.

- Incorporate Strength Training: Strength training aids in the development of lean muscle mass. Muscle burns more calories when resting, which may aid in weight loss.

Highlight Nutrient-Dense Foods:

- Choose low-calorie meals that are rich in vitamins, minerals, and satiation. Prioritize nutritious foods like vegetables, lean meats, and whole grains.

- Stay Hydrated: Hydration is essential for metabolism and hunger control. Stay hydrated by drinking lots of water throughout the day.

- Stress Management: Stress may play a role in weight loss plateaus. Stress-reduction techniques such as meditation, deep breathing, and yoga should be used.

- Get Enough Sleep: Sleep deprivation may prevent weight loss. Aim for 7-9 hours of quality sleep every night to support metabolic function.

- Keep Note of Your Progress: Keep track of your food intake, activities, and measurements. While progress may not always be visible on the scale, paying attention to other indications may help you remain motivated.

- Be Consistent and Patient: Plateaus are a normal part of the weight loss process. Maintain your dedication and focus on the long-term goal rather than the short-term fluctuations.

- Mindset Shift: Redirect your attention away from weight loss and onto other indicators of progress, such as increased energy, fitness, and happiness.

Diet Changes for Long-Term Success

To have long-term success with the Metabolic Confusion Diet, you must create good eating habits that enhance your overall health, fitness, and well-being. Here's how to make dietary changes for a long-term lifestyle change:

- Accept Balance: Strive for a nutritionally balanced diet that contains a variety of nutrient-dense foods from all food groups. Excessive restriction or overindulgence should be avoided at all costs.

- Gradual changes: Make eating changes gradually to allow your body and mind time to adjust. Changes that are quick and extreme might lead to burnout and setbacks.

- Portion control: Even while eating healthful meals, exercise portion control to prevent overeating. Use mindful eating methods to recognize hunger and fullness signals.

- Choose whole, less processed meals as your priority. These provide essential nutrients, fiber, and satiation while also encouraging long-term health.

- Include Flexibility: Treat yourself to periodic treats or indulgences in moderation. This prevents feelings of deprivation and fosters a healthy relationship with food.

- Meal Preparation: Plan your meals ahead of time to avoid making poor decisions due to a lack of time or alternatives.

- Adapt to Changes: Your diet should adapt as your goals, lifestyle, and preferences change. It should be flexible enough to accommodate different periods of your life.

- Learn from Setbacks: If you fail to stick to your diet, don't consider it a failure. Learn from your errors and go forward guilt-free.

- Drink lots of water throughout the day to stay hydrated. Hydration improves digestion, energy levels, and overall health.

- Long-term consistency is much more important than short-term greatness. Aim for a well-balanced diet most of the time.

- Consume adequate protein to enhance muscle maintenance, metabolism, and satiety.

- Address Emotional Eating: Use emotional eating management techniques such as mindfulness, stress reduction, and seeking professional assistance as needed.

- Lifelong Learning: Keep up to date on food and health problems. Understanding the science behind your eating choices may assist you in sticking to them.

- Recognize and Celebrate Successes Other Than Weight Reduction: Recognize and celebrate achievements other than weight loss, such as increased energy, strength, or improved sleep.

- Seek Help: Surround yourself with a supportive network, whether it's friends, family, or online communities where you can exchange experiences, advice, and encouragement.

- Mindset Shift: Adopt a long-term outlook. Concentrate on long-term habits rather than immediate fixes.

- Monitor Progress: Evaluate your progress frequently and adjust your plan as needed. What works at one point in your journey may need to be adjusted later.

Conclusion

The importance of a holistic approach to better health, fitness, and overall well-being cannot be overstated. Balance is a reoccurring subject in our examination of the "Metabolic Confusion Diet for Endomorphs" and the many components that contribute to its effectiveness. Long-term success involves more than just numbers on a scale; it necessitates a careful balance of diet, exercise, psychology, and lifestyle factors.

We've examined the complexity of genetics and body composition, metabolism, hormonal influences, and the special challenges that endomorphs face. We recognized the significance of macronutrient cycling, meal timing, and customization in achieving the best results. We've worked on the mental aspects of goal-setting, self-evaluation, and creating a supportive environment. We've also discussed how to cope with plateaus, emotional eating, and mental challenges.

The threads that weave this tapestry of change are patience, flexibility, and the underlying understanding that sustainable progress is a journey, not a destination. Adopting a balanced diet and lifestyle, as well as fostering a positive mindset and nurturing self-care, pave the way for long-term progress.

As we near the finish of our trip, remember that everyone's route is different, and the mix of methods that works best for you may be different. It is vital to approach this journey with compassion, considering both successes and failures as learning opportunities. Your choices today provide the framework for your future well-being, and each step toward your goals is a victory in and of itself.

As you go forward, armed with the facts and concepts we've explored, remember that change is about altering your relationship with yourself as well as your body. Accept the journey, enjoy the progress, and look forward with optimism. Your dedication to balance, consistency, and self-improvement will pave the path to a more healthy, happy, and vibrant you.

www.ingramcontent.com/pod-product-compliance
Lightning Source LLC
Chambersburg PA
CBHW060949260726
48661CB00005B/1813